Sleep Apnea Help

Learn What Sleep Apnea is and What You Need to Know About It so That You Can Deal With it Effectively and Get Happiness and Health Benefits that You Get From a Good Night's Sleep

By Nathan Weaver

© **Copyright 2019 - All rights reserved.**

The content contained within this book may not be reproduced, duplicated or transmitted without direct written permission from the author or the publisher.

Under no circumstances will any blame or legal responsibility be held against the publisher or author for any damages, reparation, or monetary loss due to the information contained within this book. Either directly or indirectly.

Legal Notice:

This book is copyright protected. This book is only for personal use. You cannot amend, distribute, sell, use, quote or paraphrase any part, or the content within this book, without the consent of the author or publisher.

Disclaimer Notice:

Please note the information contained within this document is for educational and entertainment purposes only. All effort has been executed to present accurate, up to date and reliable, complete information. No warranties of any kind are declared or implied. Readers acknowledge that the author is not engaging in the rendering of legal, financial, medical or professional advice. The content within this book has been derived from various sources. Please consult a licensed professional before attempting any techniques outlined in this book.

By reading this document, the reader agrees that under no

circumstances is the author responsible for any losses, direct or indirect, which are incurred as a result of the use of information contained within this document, including, but not limited to, —errors, omissions, or inaccuracies.

Contents

Introduction 1
Chapter 1: Classifications Of Sleep Apnea 4
    Obstructive Sleep Apnea 4
    Central Sleep Apnea 6
    Mixed or Complex Apnea 6
Chapter 2: Symptoms and Signs 8
Chapter 3: Sleep Apnea Diagnosis 13
    Physical Examinations To Check For Sleep Apnea. 18
    How Members of the Family Could Aid To Identify Sleep Apnea. 19
Chapter 4: Diagnosing Sleep Apnea 21
    Where To Locate A Sleep Specialist.. 24
Chapter 5: Kids With Sleep Apnea. 26
Chapter 6: Sleep Apnea Treatments 31
    Kinds of Treatments 31
Chapter 7: Lifestyle Modifications. 33
Chapter 8: Other Sleep Apnea Treatments 36
    CPAP (Continuous Positive Airway Pressure). 36
    Possible CPAP Side Effects 37
    Surgery 41
    Sleep Apnea Pillows 48
Chapter 9: Crucial Things About Sleep Apnea 51
Conclusion 53

Thank you for buying this book and I hope that you will find it useful. If you will want to share your thoughts on this book, you can do so by leaving a review on the Amazon page, it helps me out a lot.

Introduction

Sleep apnea is when you briefly cease breathing during sleep, or your breaths are shallow. The momentary breathing could last from a couple of seconds and go on for a couple of minutes. These breathing disruptions could occur plenty of times per hour.

Later on, you would generally breathe once again. It might be combined with loud choking or snoring. This condition could hinder you from obtaining a good night's rest. It results in you not getting as much sleep as you require. Sleep apnea induces you to be exhausted and drowsy throughout the day.

Sleep apnea is not something which is quickly diagnosed. Additionally, it is generally not discovered throughout a routine exam with your doctor. Since it occurs while you are sleeping, you most likely would not realize that you had it unless somebody sees an uncommon pattern in your sleeping.

You might find out that you have sleep apnea if somebody notices that as you are sleeping. Even then, they most likely will not understand that you might have sleep apnea.

Countless grownups are struggling with sleep apnea and do not understand it. Most of them are obese or overweight. Men struggle with sleep apnea more than ladies. The older an individual is, the more probable that they could inherit sleep apnea. With ladies, they could develop this condition in the post-menopausal phase.

Minority groups, like Hispanics, African-Americans and Pacific Islanders develop this condition more than other ethnic groups. It could additionally be inherited from members of the family. If you have little air passages in your throat, nose or mouth, you are more prone to having this condition.

Young kids that have bigger than regular tonsil tissues could additionally establish sleep apnea. You could additionally be at risk for sleep apnea if you:

- Have hypertension.

- Smoke.

- Heart Failure

- Potential for having a stroke.

Chapter 1: Classifications Of Sleep Apnea

There are 3 kinds of sleep apnea, yet just 2 are discussed the most. There is obstructive sleep apnea, and that is the most frequent kind of sleep apnea. With obstructive sleep apnea, your throat muscles collapse as you're sleeping.

The other kind of sleep apnea is referred to as central sleep apnea. This kind occurs when your breathing muscles do not get the appropriate signals. The third one, that many folks do not experience, is referred to as mixed or complex sleep apnea. This kind is a mix of both conditions.

Obstructive Sleep Apnea

Obstructive sleep apnea, or OSA, obstructs the throat's air passage. Certain other things which occur with this kind of sleep disorder are:

- Air is going to pass through the upper airway. This consists of the nose, throat and mouth areas.

- As you're sleeping, the muscles of the throat collapse inward during breathing.

- You are going to have less oxygen in your blood. This induces your lungs to take in air from the outside.

- As the muscles become broader, they obstruct the collapse for the airway to stay open.

- Even when you make snorting sounds or gasp for air, you might not always get up.

- Apnea occurs when the back throat tissues are momentarily obstructed. You cease breathing, and if you get up, you might need to gasp for breath.

In case you encounter 5 or more apnea episodes per hour, it is seen as an aspect of obstructive sleep apnea.

Central Sleep Apnea

Central sleep apnea is not as frequent as obstructive sleep apnea. This kind of sleep apnea begins in the brain. The brain is not going to send a signal to the airway muscles to ensure that they are able breathe.

The oxygen level declines, and you are going to most likely wake up. With this kind of sleep apnea, individuals typically remember waking up. In case you have heart disease or cardiac arrest, then you are encountering central sleep apnea.

Mixed or Complex Apnea

As pointed out previously, this is the mix of central and obstructive sleep apnea. With this kind of sleep apnea, you are going to deal with obstructive sleep apnea, or OSA. Along with that, with good airway pressure, you are going to have continual central sleep apnea.

In case you are utilizing CPAP (Continuous Positive Airway Pressure), the central sleep apnea is going to be acknowledged. This occurs after the obstruction has actually been cleared.

Chapter 2: Symptoms and Signs

The most apparent symptom of sleep apnea is constant and loud snoring. You might pause during snoring. You might additionally gasp or choke after pausing. Whenever you sleep on your rear, the snoring becomes louder. In case you sleep on your side, the snoring might not be as loud.

You might or might not snore each night. Ultimately, the snoring might increase, and it might become more loud as you sleep.

Considering that you're sleeping while you're gasping or snoring, you might not realize that you're experiencing breathing problems. Others are going to see the indications ahead of you and are going to let you know if it ends up being a pattern. Understand that just because you might be a chronic snorer, it does not indicate that you have sleep apnea.

If you are dealing with sleep throughout the day, that may be an indication of sleep apnea. If you're not a part of any activity, you might wind up going to sleep really rapidly. If this occurs when you're driving or at work, the odds are higher that you might wind up in a work-related accident or an accident as you're driving.

There are other symptoms and signs which individuals might not connect with sleep apnea. They are:

- Regular urination in the night or evening hours

- Headaches in the early morning

- Can't focus, concentrate or memory loss

- Moodiness or feeling a change in your character

- Dry throat in the early morning as you get up

Your throat muscles are utilized to maintain the airway open to ensure that you could get air into your lungs. Nevertheless, during sleeping, your muscles of the throat are relaxed. This suggests that your airway could be obstructed, and air will not enter into your lungs.

With obstructive sleep apnea, you could additionally experience these:

- In case you have a small structure at the neck and head, the airway size might be tinier in your throat and mouth.

- Being obese or overweight, you are going to have extra soft fat tissue. This tissue could become thick in the windpipe wall. There is very little of an opening, and what is out there might not remain open.

- Your throat muscles and your tongue muscles are more relaxed than they ought to be.

- With the obstructed air passages, you might wind up snoring loudly as you sleep.

- In case you are an older grownup, your brain signals might not maintain the your throat muscles stiff as they ought to.

Low levels of oxygen make you incapable of gettinga good night's sleep. The muscles in the upper air passage become tight, and your windpipe is open. You have the ability to breathe ordinarily again until you begin choking or snorting.

Together with the frequent low oxygen levels and fewer hours of sleep, your stress hormones are discharged. This may cause you to have hypertension, a stroke, cardiac arrest and irregular heartbeats. The stress hormones could additionally lead to you having a cardiac arrest.

If your condition is not dealt with, you might be at a higher risk of diabetes and obesity.

Chapter 3: Sleep Apnea Diagnosis

The manner in which doctors diagnose sleep apnea depends upon family and medical histories. They are going to additionally carry out a physical exam. They are going to examine your signs. If they feel that the indications, signs and patterns fit this condition, then you are going to be referred for a sleep study.

Sleep studies are measurements which reveal your sleeping pattern. The outcomes demonstrate how well and how much you sleep. If you have any issues with your sleeping, the studies are going to reveal the outcomes of that.

In case you are referred for a sleep study, it is essential that you get one. The study could figure out if you have actually been diagnosed with a sleep disorder, like sleep apnea. Sleep apnea and other sleep disorders could boost your health risk for strokes, hypertension and cardiac arrest.

Physicians experienced in reading sleep studies could quickly detect sleep apnea and supply treatment to ensure that you are able to sleep better during the night. The essential thing is to allow your doctor know about any unfavorable sleeping habits you have dealt with.

They would entail tiredness and chronic drowsiness throughout the day. Additionally, advise your doctor if you have actually had trouble going to sleep or getting up during the night and can't return to sleep.

You may be struggling with a sleep disorder which you aren't aware of. Physicians with experience in sleep disorders are going to ask you about your sleep schedule. They are going to additionally ask your members of the family about any chronic snoring which they have actually handled.

Physicians with experience in sleep disorders are referred to as sleep specialists. They could quickly identify and supply the treatment for people dealing with issues sleeping.

So as to assist the specialists in identifying what's happening, you ought to establish and maintain a sleep journal for no more than 2 weeks. This is the start of the sleep study. Here are certain questions which you might see in a sleep journal:

- The time you went to sleep the night before

- The number of hours you slept the night before

- The time you got up in the morning

- How long did it take you to drop off to sleep the night before

- The number of times you got up throughout the night

- If you were drowsy when you got up in the morning

- Which meds you took the night before

- The amount of beverages you had throughout the day

- The number of drinks with caffeine you had throughout the day

- How many naps you had

- The time when you drank the alcoholic drinks

- If you were really drowsy throughout the day

- The length of those naps

- If you were relatively alert throughout the day

- If you were a bit tired throughout the day

- If you were wide awake throughout the day

Your doctor might additionally inquire about the following:

- Gasping.

- Snorting.

- Morning headaches

If the results of the journal point to:

- Waking up more than a couple of times throughout the night.

- Regular naps.

- Continuously being drowsy in the daytime.

- Needing more than a half-hour to fall sleep.

Physical Examinations To Check For Sleep Apnea.

Throughout the physical examination, your doctor is going to examine the areas of your throat, mouth and nose. They are going to be trying to find enlarged or extra tissues. For kids diagnosed with sleep apnea, they generally have enlarged tonsils. With them, it does not take a lot to give a medical diagnosis aside from an examination and medical history.

For grownups, the doctors try to find an enlarged uvula, a bit of tissue which hangs and sits from the middle of the rear of your mouth. They additionally search for a soft palate, which remains in the rear of your throat and is referred to as the roof of your mouth in that place.

How Members of the Family Could Aid To Identify Sleep Apnea.

Due to the fact that many people do not understand that they're struggling with sleep apnea, it is essential that there is somebody who is able to identify irregularities while you sleep. The individual does not know that their breathing could begin and stop at any time throughout the night. They additionally do not take into account when somebody tells them that they are loud and chronic snorer.

There are things which members of the family may do to assist:

- Telling them to consult their doctor.

- Letting a member of the family understand that they have a chronic loud snoring case.

- Being there for them emotionally. This could be a tough time for them, and they require all of the assistance that they are able to get.

- In case they are diagnosed with sleep apnea, advising them to abide by directions, consisting of any post-op, treatments and follow-up.

Chapter 4: Diagnosing Sleep Apnea

Sleep studies are generally carried out in a sleep center or a sleep laboratory. This might or might not be in a medical facility. If the study is performed in the sleep center, you might have an overnight stay. Nevertheless, this is not constantly engraved in stone.

The beneficial thing about sleep studies is that you are not going to feel any discomfort. The one thing which might impact you is skin irritation from the sensors. When the sensing units are removed from your skin, you are not going to deal with any more irritation.

Even though the risks of sleep studies are marginal, these studies require some time (at least a couple of hours).

There are various tests for sleep studies. One of them is referred to as a polysomnogram or PSG test. This test is performed in a sleep center or sleep laboratory. More than probably, with this test, an overnight stay will be required.

You are going to have electrodes and monitors on your scalp, face, chest, limbs and fingers. As you are sleeping, the following things are going to be monitored:

- Your brain activity

- The motion of your eyes

- The pace of your heart

- Your muscle activity

- Blood pressure

- The tempo of your heart

- The amount of oxygen in your blood

- Air motion in and out of your lungs

As you sleep, the staff on duty are going to utilize sensors to examine your as you sleep throughout the night. After the PSG is done, the sleep expert is going to go over the results with you. They are going to have the ability to identify whether you have sleep apnea and if it is a problem or not. From the results, they are going to have the ability to chart a course of treatment.

A Multiple Sleep Latency Test or MSLT is utilized to identify how drowsy you are during the daytime. This test is generally carried out after a PSG. You are going to have devices put on your scalp for monitoring reasons.

With this test, you are going to need to take at least 5 naps, each lasting 20 minutes. This ought to be carried out every 2 hours throughout times when you would be alert. The testers are going to examine how long it is going to require you to go to sleep and how long you slept.

Those individuals who take less than 5 minutes to get to sleep are more probable prospects for a sleep disorder. When the screening is carried out, the sleep specialist is going to supply you with the results and talk to you about options for treatment.

Where To Locate A Sleep Specialist

If you require help discovering a sleep specialist, there are a number of organizations which could help you with that, like:

- American Academy of Sleep Medicine (AASM)

- American Academy of Dental Sleep Medicine (AADSM)

- American Board of Sleep Medicine (ABSM)

These organizations are comprised of doctors, scientists and dentists who work with individuals impacted with this sleep disorder. They work to additionally the development of sleep research and sleep medicine.

The doctors and researchers who serve on the relevant boards are noted as "Board Certified" in the sleep medicine niche. The ABSM maintains an updated sleep specialist listing. They could be found by the state or by their name. The AADSM maintains an updated dentist listing who focus on dealing with sleep apnea patients by utilizing oral devices.

Chapter 5: Kids With Sleep Apnea.

Kids diagnosed with sleep apnea could be aggressive and hyperactive. They could additionally suffer considerably in their studies. Often they might sleep in a different way than ordinary. They might additionally wet the bed. Throughout the daytime hours, a few of them are going to breathe through their mouth rather than their nose.

Loudly snoring, gasping for air, snorting, and momentary stoppage in breathing all are indications of sleep apnea. Essentially, their symptoms and signs are parallel with what grownups have.

Even with this, doctors can not constantly spot this sleep disorder in kids. They figure that it's not a big deal due to the fact that most of them are hyperactive anyhow.

There are certain things which you might do to discover if your kid, in fact, has sleep apnea:

- Talk to your kid's pediatrician and allow them to understand what's happening.

- Talk to an ENT (ear, nose and throat) specialist.

- Talk to a pulmonologist (lung specialist) specializing in kids.

- Psychiatrists, psychologists and other medical providers could additionally aid with a medical diagnosis.

If you have medical insurance, make certain to talk to them initially to see if you require referrals for particular medical providers.

If there is additional testing to be carried out, check to see if the doctors are board-certified to deal with kids with sleep apnea. Do not hesitate to inquire about their credentials. Besides, this is your kid's health that you're handling. With them, any medical diagnosis could need delicate care and consideration.

The doctor is going to additionally have to know if they are taking medications and if the kid is allergic to anything. Additionally, advise them of any problems with their habits and development. Along with that, supply them with information on their nighttime sleep patterns and if they take naps.

The kid might need to take a sleep study or polysomnogram (PSG) to identify the seriousness of their sleep apnea. There are other tests which are given to make a determination. They consist of:

- An electrooculogram (EOG), that is utilized for eye and chin measurements;

- An electroencephalogram (EEG), that is utilized to assess the brain wave activity;

- Tests utilizing chest bands for breathing motion measurements;

- An electrocardiogram (EKG), that is utilized for tempo and heart rate measurements;

- Tests utilizing more monitors for oxygen levels and levels of co2 in the kid's blood.

Most of the sleep studies for kids call for an overnight stay. There are not a great deal of medical facilities which focus on sleep apnea for kids. Even with that, the ones which are utilized for grownups are going to use them to test kids too.

Check the facility to learn if they work with kids who might have this sleep disorder. Just like grownups, check different groups and organizations to locate a certified sleep specialist.

Additionally, similar to grownups, if sleep apnea goes without treatment in kids, they could additionally experience severe health problems down the road. Kids could additionally worsen with their behavioral patterns and academics in school if they are not dealt with promptly. Do not take for granted that they might simply be going through a tough time when it might be sleep apnea.

Chapter 6: Sleep Apnea Treatments

The function of dealing with sleep apnea (obstructive) is to enable the patient to be capable of breathing routinely as they sleep. The treatment additionally aids in getting alleviation from loudly snoring and being chronically drowsy throughout the day.

Sleep apnea treatment additionally aids in decreasing medical issues, like diabetes, heart disease, hypertension and other medical conditions.

Kinds of Treatments

There are various kinds of treatments to utilize for sleep apnea. Here are a few of the more typical ones:

- CPAP.

- Lifestyle modifications

- Surgery.

- Mouthpiece or oral appliance.

- Therapies.

With treatment, you could obtain more sleep and do away with being tired and drowsy throughout the daytime. Your general health is going to improve together with you being happier that you have the ability to sleep more without being interrupted during the night.

It could additionally help the person sleeping next to you to get more sleep too. You will not be interrupting them by waking up at various times of the night, making gasping and snorting noises.

Chapter 7: Lifestyle Modifications.

In case you sleep on your rear, you are subject to establishing sleep apnea. How you set up yourself as you lie down on the bed could make or break you. It could determine the number of times you encounter obstructive sleep apnea. It additionally determines how moderate or severe sleep apnea could impact you.

In some cases, it has to do with gravity. Gravity could cause your throat not to obtain ample air when you are resting on your back. Those who sleep on their backs could experience as much as 80 apneas per hour. They could do away with this problem by sleeping either on their left or right side. Nevertheless, if you are obese or overweight, this might not assist a lot.

You could make certain lifestyle modifications so as to take care of central and obstructive sleep apnea:

- If you are obese or overweight, dropping weight could assist. Weight loss could assist your throat to be less limiting. Eat more healthy vegetables and fruits. Be more active physically. If you are unsure how to set about weight loss, talk to your doctor.

- Leave the sleeping tablets and related medicines alone. Additionally, do not consume alcohol as a sedative to get you to sleep.

- Your nasal passageway must not be obstructed. If you have difficulty maintaining them open, utilize a nasal stick or spray. You could additionally utilize decongestants, yet it's not for long-lasting usage.

- In case you are accustomed to sleeping on your back, that could be an issue. Attempt sleeping on your stomach or your side. If you sleep on your back, your tongue and soft palate of your throat are going to sit on the back. This generates an obstruction of the throat's airway.

- Raise the head of your bed to boost your oxygen levels which you're ingesting.

- If you smoke, you are going to need to quit as soon as you can.

Alternative treatments, like acupuncture, have been utilized to deal with sleep apnea, yet there is more research to be done. Due to this, do not utilize this technique as a way to get rid of this condition. Speak with your doctor prior to thinking about any alternative sleep apnea treatment.

Chapter 8: Other Sleep Apnea Treatments

If lifestyle modifications do not aid in treating your sleep apnea, then your case is more serious than what you initially believed. Here are certain other treatments which might aid:

CPAP (Continuous Positive Airway Pressure).

CPAP (Continuous Positive Airway Pressure) is a technique where a machine generates air pressure. So as to get it, you need to put on a mask. The mask is positioned on your nose as you're sleeping.

When you are utilizing CPAP, you get more air pressure than you would if you were simply breathing in the outside air. The air pressure with this machine assists in keeping your upper airway passageways open. This aids in preventing apnea and snoring.

Initially, not everybody who utilizes this machine is going to feel comfy with it. Due to how it's made, it might not feel right in the beginning. Nevertheless, with modifications and making the straps fit appropriately, you are going to have the ability to get accustomed to donning it.

Nevertheless, if the mask you have is not settling in, then you might need to discover another one. Along with that, you could utilize a humidifier in addition to the CPAP for extra comfort.

There might be times when you have other issues. Nevertheless, do not stop utilizing it. Rather, check with your doctor to see what could be done and make extra adjustments or corrections. If you have actually put on weight, the air pressure settings need to be modified.

Possible CPAP Side Effects

Throughout the initial couple of nights that you don this device, it may get on your nerves due to the fact that it is not immediately comfortable to wear. It makes you wish to stop sleep apnea treatment.

Nevertheless, it would defeat the purpose. You could utilize the low air pressure device at first.

The majority of people who utilize CPAP claim that they experience side effects. The majority of them are managing the mask itself. You could pick a mask which offers comfort and stops it from leaking a great deal of air pressure.

Here are a few of the side effects which you might experience with the device:

- More air pressure than ordinary-- you could have a tough time breathing out when that takes place.

- Irritated eyes.

- Throat and nose irritation.

- Experiencing upper respiratory area infections if you do not maintain the device tidy.

- Sore mouth.

- Dry mouth.

- Nose sores from putting on the device too firmly.

- Blockage in the nasal area.

- Chest muscles discomfort

There are going to be other times when the CPAP is going to need to be calibrated. Your doctor or a sleep specialist could show you how to do this. As soon as you discover how to do it, you are going to have the ability to save cash by not needing to make visits to see your doctor or specialist (unless absolutely required).

You could additionally get devices which are going to aid you to get more air in your throat. They can be adjusted and are created to fit your requirements so as to get more air flowing through your throat.

The tool calibrates the air pressure as you're sleeping. You do not need to press a button or utilize a dial to adjust it. The adjustment is made instantly as you sleep.

An oral appliance or a mouthpiece is an additional option if the CPAP does not get the job done for you. This device is utilized to maintain your throat open to ensure that you can get air. It could assist those encountering moderate sleep apnea.

Despite the fact that the CPAP is more helpful than the mouthpiece, the latter has actually been proven more convenient for certain individuals to utilize while they're sleeping. It opens your throat by moving your lower jaw forward. Doing this could aid your snoring and treat moderate obstructive sleep apnea.

You could get a mouthpiece from a dental practitioner. It might take time to locate the ideal one which you could be comfy with. It is necessary that you talk to the dentist each 6 months after you begin using it.

After the initial year of wearing, you could talk to the dentist once a year. You wish to ensure that it is still fitting right and functioning correctly. If you are feeling any pain, do not be reluctant to call the dentist for a potential adjustment.

Surgery

Surgery is one more alternative to utilize so as to deal with sleep apnea. With the surgery, extra tissue is extracted from your throat or nose. This procedure is just carried out in a hospital.

One more alternative is to stiffen or shrink the extra tissue or the lower jaw could be reset. When the tissue is being stiffened or shrunk, the treatment is typically carried out in a doctor's office or in a hospital.

If the shrinking treatment is carried out, you might need to get a couple of shots in the tissue area. If the excess tissue has to be shrunk additionally, you might require other treatments besides the shots. Additionally, the stiffening process consists of the doctor creating a little cut in the excess tissue and putting a little bit of plastic that is stiff.

Throughout the pre-surgery, you are going to be administered a bit of medicine which is to make you go to sleep. So, throughout the surgery, you are going to be out and not feel anything up until you awaken. When the surgery is carried out in the hospital, you might experience throat pain lasting between 7 days and 14 days.

Here are certain surgical options to deal with sleep apnea and aid you to rest better:

- UPPP (Uvulopalatopharyngoplasty) This is a treatment where tissue is extracted from the rear of your mouth. The tissue is additionally taken out from the top part of your throat. Along with getting rid of tissue, your adenoids and tonsils are additionally taken out.

With this surgery, your snoring might stop; nevertheless, considering that there is still tissue further down in your throat, it is not likely that it is going to cure or treat your sleep apnea. With the tissue staying there, your airway is closed. With UPPP surgical treatment, you are going to need to heading to a hospital for a surgery.

With this surgical treatment, you are going to experience a great deal of pain. You are going to be recovering for numerous weeks. This surgery is just carried out on individuals experiencing serious obstructive sleep apnea. Even then, there are just some who undergo this treatment.

This is not one of those surgeries where you can get up, and it's back to business. If you have the ability to have the UPPP surgery, you might run the risk of certain complications, such as:

- Your throat might get infected if no antibiotics are provided before the surgical treatment.

- The throat muscles and soft palate might not work correctly.

- You might experience fluids coming up through your nose or mouth.

- You might have issues swallowing.

- You might not have the ability to smell.

It is not guaranteed that surgery will make you feel better. You might still have a reoccurrence of episodes of sleep apnea. Even utilizing CPAP is not going to be as helpful after the surgery. There are certain oral surgeries which could be carried out:

- A tracheostomy-- this surgery is carried out if previous treatments did not assist you. It is additionally utilized if your sleep apnea is serious to the point where it's a question of life or death.

From your neck opening, a tube created from plastic or metal is put in and utilized for you to breathe from. The opening remains covered in the daytime and exposed during the night. You require air to go in and out of your lungs as you sleep.

- Maxillomandibular advancement-- This surgery is utilized to prevent blockage of your throat by making the space bigger where your soft palate and tongue are located.

The lower and upper part of your jaw is moved toward the front. This is how the enlargement is produced. This procedure is complicated, and an orthodontist and oral surgeon might need to do it together.

Surgeons utilize lasers to do away with unneeded tissues in the rear of your throat. They could additionally utilize radiofrequency energy. Both of these procedures are great to utilize for dealing with snoring. Although they could be utilized to alleviate snoring, they must not be utilized to deal with obstructive sleep apnea.

There are more procedures which are utilized to alleviate snoring. A few of them could aid with dealing with sleep apnea. Nevertheless, the procedures are not cures for this sleep condition.

They consist of:

- Removing enlarged tonsils or adenoids

- Nasal surgery-- polyps are taken out, or a partition placed in between your nostrils is straightened out.

Extra surgical procedures which are utilized might deal with irregularities on your face. There are additionally surgical procedures for extra blockages. Both of these could cause you to have sleep apnea. The procedures could be carried out solo or together.

Other surgeries include:

- Plastic chin surgery

- Hyoid surgery-- the bone beneath the chin which could move is moved toward the front. As it moves, the tongue muscle moves along with it.

- Tongue advancement-- this procedure entails a cut at the crossway of the tongue and jawbone.

Having surgery to deal with apnea is not a certainty. It depends upon what type of surgery it is and the particulars of the sleep apnea.

For complex and central sleep apnea, various therapies could be utilized. A few of them are:

- Medical treatments for neuromuscular problems.

- CPAP (Continuous Positive Airway Pressure).

- BiPAP (Bilevel Positive Airway Pressure)-- This is when greater pressure is utilized for breathing in. When you breathe out, the air pressure becomes lower. This aids in reinforcing your breathing pattern if you have central sleep apnea. The device could be set to automatic mode if it spots that you have not breathed into it after a couple of seconds.

- ASV (Adaptive servo-ventilation)-- This is a new airflow device which gets a taste of how you breathe ordinarily. It maintains your information about your breathing pattern in a computer.

As long as you're sleeping, the ASV functions to maintain your breathing pattern at an ordinary rate and to get rid of any breathing pauses. In case you have central sleep apnea, this technique might work better for you than CPAP.

Sleep Apnea Pillows

There are certain individuals who do get the advised quantity of sleep, yet they still get up tired. This could be linked to their snoring. Snoring is a really serious medical concern. To deal with that, sleep apnea pillows could be utilized.

Sleep apnea pillows have actually been recognized to deal with sleep apnea in certain individuals. Before you attempt one, you need to understand whether you are simply snoring or if the snoring is an outcome of obstructive sleep apnea.

Sleep apnea pillows could aid the airway of your throat to remain open. Due to the fact that sleep apnea causes your breathing to be uneven and disrupted, the pillow functions to make your breathing regular again. The uneven and disrupted breathing typically occurs throughout the night when you are sleeping.

The special pillows are developed with foam panels which are elevated, unlike a normal pillow. The elevation functions to maintain your head slanted. This aids to boost your breathing pattern to render it regular and undisturbed once again.

Sleep apnea pillows could be created to where they could be utilized in more than one sleeping position. They are flexible so that you could sleep in a manner in which is most comfy for you. They offer you with a great deal of assistance to ensure that you could get a good night's sleep.

The sleep apnea pillow additionally assists in these ways regarding sleep apnea:

- Supplies comfort and assistance to ensure that you could obtain a good night's sleep

- Obstructed airways are opened-- this aids with sleep apnea and snoring relief

- The pillow enables you to sleep like a newborn

- Alleviates you from the fatigue which you feel due to your sleep apnea

There are individuals who are chronic snorers who have actually never utilized these kinds of pillows and do not wish to have a go at them. They would prefer to get sleeping tablets and wind up becoming dependent on them. Medication is not a great alternative to help you with sleep apnea or snoring. Actually, medication is not advised since it has actually proven not to be helpful.

Chapter 9: Crucial Things About Sleep Apnea

Here are certain essential points which you ought to understand about sleep apnea:

- Sleep apnea is a chronic condition wherein your sleep is disrupted more than 3 nights weekly.

- Obstructive sleep apnea is the most frequent of the 3 that are pointed out.

- Due to the fact that snoring is ordinary for certain individuals, this sleep disorder could be easily be ignored.

- If you are obese or overweight and struggling with sleep apnea, work on dropping weight. When you do, do not put the pounds back on.

- Being chronically sleepy in the daytime could lead to you having a work-related mishap.

- There are various ways to get sleep apnea treatment. Based upon the intensity of your condition, the sleep specialist and the doctor are going to work to get the most effective treatment for you.

- A member of the family could determine something might be wrong when the individual is choking and gasping for air and not obtaining ample sleep.

- Kids that have behavioral issues and problems with academics are frequently ignored. These indications are typically not linked with sleep apnea.

- Individuals must not make fun of those who are struggling with sleep apnea. This is a really considerable sleep condition which needs to be treated urgently.

Conclusion

Sleep apnea is a condition where the signs are not quickly acknowledged. Nevertheless, down the line, somebody might observe something. Bear in mind that even if your snoring might be chronic, it's not a certainty that you are dealing with a sleep disorder. The only manner in which you'll find out is with sleep studies and examinations.

It is essential that if you or somebody else suspects something suspicious in your sleeping pattern, that you speak with a doctor as soon as you can. It might just ensure that you receive treatment in time to protect against significant health problems.

I hope that you enjoyed reading through this book and that you have found it useful. If you want to share your thoughts on this book, you can do so by leaving a review on the Amazon page. Have a great rest of the day.

Printed in Great Britain
by Amazon